NATIONAL VISIT 2

A visit by the Mental Health Act Commission to 104 mental health and learning disability units in England and Wales.

Improving Care for Detained Patients from Black and Minority Ethnic Communities. PRELIMINARY REPORT

Lesley Warner   Sarala Nicholas   Kamlesh Patel   Jennifer Harris   Richard Ford

How society relates to those of its members from minority ethnic groups is a measure of its values and standards. Nowhere is this more relevant than in the provision of health and social care for those with mental health problems – especially under compulsion.

This report of the Mental Health Act Commission's Second National Visit describes important aspects of the care and treatment of black and minority ethnic detained patients in England and Wales, and identifies the considerable progress that remains to be made in order to achieve a standard of service that is both acceptable and nationally consistent. The report also provides examples of good practice which are making a real contribution to the achievement of the ultimate goal – that good practice becomes common practice.

I hope that people from black and minority ethnic communities with an interest in the treatment of mental health problems, the commissioners and providers of mental health services and those responsible for providing the strategic and policy framework for the delivery of those services, will find this report both informative and helpful.

Gordon H Lakes CB, MC
MHAC Chairman 1998–1999

ACKNOWLEDGEMENTS

The methodology for the Mental Health Act Commission's Second National Visit was devised, and the data analysed, by:

- **Lesley Warner,** *Senior Researcher,* The Sainsbury Centre for Mental Health

- **Sarala Nicholas,** *Statistician,* The Sainsbury Centre for Mental Health

- **Kamlesh Patel,** *Director of the Ethnicity and Health Unit,* University of Central Lancashire

- **Jennifer Harris,** *formerly Principal Lecturer, Ethnicity and Health Unit,* University of Central Lancashire

- **Richard Ford,** *Head of Service Evaluation,* The Sainsbury Centre for Mental Health

We would like to thank the Team Managers, Commissioners, and other staff of the Mental Health Act Commission, who were responsible for the organisation of the Second National Visit, contributed to the development of the questionnaire, carried out pilot interviews, and undertook the Visit. Special thanks are due to William Bingley, Chief Executive, Cheryl Robinson, Director of Finance and Operations, Ruth Runciman, former Chairman, and Peter Stace of the Secretariat.

We are very grateful to the managers and staff of all the units visited for their co-operation and assistance with the Second National Visit, and to all those who provided us with copies of their written policies, procedures and guidelines.

Finally, we would like to thank all the units which allowed us to pilot early versions of the questionnaire, enabling us to modify and refine it:

- **Calderdale NHS Trust**

- **Kirklees NHS Trust**

- **North Essex Mental Health NHS Trust**

- **North West London Mental Health NHS Trust (now part of Brent, Kensington, Chelsea and Westminster Mental Health NHS Trust)**

- **Nottingham Healthcare Trust**

- **Rampton Hospital Authority**

- **Retford Lodge**

- **Riverside Mental Health Services NHS Trust (now part of Brent, Kensington, Chelsea and Westminster Mental Health NHS Trust)**

- **Surrey Oaklands NHS Trust**

- **West London Healthcare NHS Trust (now part of Ealing, Hammersmith and Fulham NHS Trust)**

SUMMARY

The Visit

- The Mental Health Act Commission, within the context of its equality strategy and following the First National Visit in 1996, undertook a Second National Visit on 11 May 1999, in collaboration with The Sainsbury Centre for Mental Health, and the Ethnicity and Health Unit at the University of Central Lancashire.

- Commissioners and Secretariat staff (hereafter referred to as Visitors) conducted the visits, mostly in pairs, to a sample of inpatient units for people aged primarily between 16 and 65 in England and Wales.

- The Visit focused on the care of black and minority ethnic detained patients, specifically looking at: ethnic monitoring, dealing with racial harassment of patients, staff training in race equality and anti-discriminatory practice, and the provision of, access to, and use of interpreters.

- 104 mental health and learning disability units were visited. These included acute and medium secure units, and high secure hospitals in the NHS, and acute and medium secure facilities in the independent sector.

- Information was collected from 119 wards, and from the case notes of 534 black and minority ethnic detained patients.

- The presence of written policies cannot be taken as proof of good practice, nor does their absence necessarily denote poor practice; however, they indicate that an issue has at least been considered. The Visit explored practice in the units and wards, to determine to what extent the policies were being followed.

The patients

- The largest minority ethnic group among the patients was Black Caribbean, comprising 42% of the total. More than two thirds of the patients were men, and the majority were aged between 25 and 44 years.

- 116 patients did not have English as their first language; between them they spoke 26 different languages. Fluency in English varied between nearly all of the Black Caribbean patients to only half of the Bangladeshi patients.

- The most commonly recorded religion was Christianity, with Muslims comprising the next largest group.

Recording and monitoring ethnicity

- Since 1995, NHS Trusts have been required to record the ethnicity of all patients admitted; this is also mandatory for independent sector units providing care to NHS-funded patients.

- Half the units had written policies, procedures or guidelines on recording ethnicity of patients. All units routinely recorded patients' ethnicity, but not all used the ONS categories. With a few exceptions, this data is not being put to great use.

- In order to draw up a package of care which takes account of a patient's ethnic, cultural and communication needs, it is necessary to accurately collect and clearly record information on ethnicity, language, dialect and religion.

- Without knowing the language and dialect spoken by their patients, ward staff will be unable to obtain an appropriate interpreter. The interrelationship between language, dialect and religion demonstrates the importance of recording full information on all of these.

Dealing with racial harassment of black and minority ethnic patients by other patients, or by staff

- Three-quarters of the units had no policy on dealing with racial harassment of black and minority ethnic patients by other patients, or by staff. Fifty-nine patients (11%) whose notes were examined had reported incidents of racial harassment.

- We were disappointed to see so few policies on racial harassment on the wards. However, the quality of those which were presented to Visitors was high.

Training in race equality and anti-discriminatory practice

- Two thirds of the units had no policy on training in race equality and anti-discriminatory practice for staff, and a similar number did not provide training on this for their staff. However, several examples of good practice were provided, demonstrating a wide range of training and other activities aimed at raising staff's awareness and understanding of the religious and cultural needs of black and minority ethnic patients. Many units had devised resource packs containing useful information.

- Although there were some signs that staffs' training needs were beginning to be addressed, this was happening in only a minority of units. Good practice will only become ingrained when all units have policies which are fully implemented so that all staff have received training.

Provision of, access to and use of interpreters

- Half the units had a policy on the provision and use of interpreters, but only three-quarters used interpreters who were trained in interpreting. Not all unit managers knew if the interpreters they used were trained in interpreting, or if they had received any mental health training.

- Half the wards had a policy on accessing and using interpreters. Although most ward managers said their staff were not trained in the use of interpreters, about two thirds said they spent time with an interpreter before an interview and in debriefing afterwards, both of which indicate good practice.

- Two thirds of the wards had used patients' relatives or friends to interpret for them; this is of concern, as widespread use of family members as interpreters can compromise objective decision-making by staff.

- Although most ward managers said that patients could request an interpreter, only a third of these could recall this happening. It is worrying that only 31 of the 56 patients not fluent in English had ever used an interpreter.

- Although people from black and minority ethnic groups may be fluent in English, at times of stress, including periods of mental illness, some may prefer to use their mother tongue and would therefore require an interpreter.

Conclusions

- One immediate effect of the Visit, and of the many pilot visits which preceded it, has been to raise the awareness of many units to the specific issues in caring for this group of patients, which is a necessary precursor to any change in practice.

- The Visit has shown that there is still a considerable development agenda. People from black and minority ethnic communities are often not receiving care that is sensitive to their cultural backgrounds. This is reflected in the Visit's findings on recording and monitoring of ethnicity, harassment, training of staff and use of interpreters.

- The aims of the Visit were to raise awareness of the issues, and to improve care for detained patients from black and minority ethnic groups. Further analysis of the data, as well as a thorough examination of all the written policies and procedures collected from the units and wards visited, will identify further examples of good practice which can be disseminated, to help those services which have been slower to develop in these areas.

- Some excellent examples of good practice have already been identified, and there will be further dissemination to share our findings, so that good practice becomes common practice. Additionally, service commissioners and providers may want to use some of the methods used in the National Visit for ongoing audit.

INTRODUCTION

Since its inception, The Mental Health Act Commission (MHAC) has been concerned about the care and treatment of patients from black and minority ethnic groups detained under the Mental Health Act 1983. The Commission's first Biennial Report (1985) highlighted significant issues in relation to patients from black and minority ethnic communities detained under the Mental Health Act (1983). Specifically, it stated that:

- **people from black and minority ethnic communities suffered disadvantages additional to those commonly experienced by mentally ill people;**

- **people from black and minority ethnic communities are detained disproportionately and in some cases inappropriately;**

- **the lack of Commissioners from these communities further compounded the situation.**

The following six Biennial Reports continued to highlight a broad range of inequalities that exist with respect to the care and treatment of black and minority ethnic detained patients.

The seventh Biennial Report (1997) summed up the position: *'Provision for patients from minority ethnic communities often remains basic, insensitive and piecemeal, leading to patients feeling alienated and isolated. It is dispiriting that the serious issues of inappropriate care and treatment of patients from black and minority ethnic communities, which were raised in previous Biennial Reports, continue to cause concern and to be noted in reports of Commission Visits'.*

Over the years, the Commission has suggested many policy and practice measures, including the provision of translated leaflets, the provision of appropriately sensitive environments taking into account patients' dietary, religious and cultural backgrounds, and women-only environments. Although some of these measures have met with positive change, service development in these areas remains *ad hoc*, patchy and piecemeal. The issues of ethnic monitoring, provision of, access to and use of interpreters, and racial harassment, have been consistently raised as matters requiring urgent attention.

The Commission recognised that it is clearly not enough merely to comment year on year about the continuing poor practice witnessed in relation to minority ethnic detained patients. The need to develop and implement a more pro-active strategy to tackle these fundamental issues of inequality was evident. The Commission was also well aware that it could not expect other agencies to provide services founded upon principles of equality without demonstrating that it had incorporated such principles into its own policies and practices.

To this end the MHAC Management Board took the decision to have a comprehensive examination of equality issues within the Commission. It recognised that it needed a clear vision statement and a long-term realistic implementation programme. The Commission did not simply want to incorporate an existing equality statement without a clear examination of the reasons, concerns and benefits of so doing.

After careful consideration and discussion the MHAC adopted and published its Equal Opportunities Policy Statement together with a set of clear goals, identifying clear areas of implementation.

A phased strategic implementation plan of inter-related activities, phase 1 being three years, set out both short- and long-term goals concerning staffing (including training) and policy and practice issues addressing the five key goals set.

Within the context of this equality strategy, and following on from the successful First National Visit in 1996[1] which included an assessment of the care of women patients, a Second National Visit was planned to address the key areas of ethnic monitoring, racial harassment, staff training and interpreters, which were recurring areas of concern to the MHAC. By identifying the current situation, and highlighting particular problems and how these have been overcome in some areas, the Commission aimed to contribute to the improvement of the care provided. As in the First National Visit, the Commission worked in collaboration with The Sainsbury Centre for Mental Health, and additionally with the Ethnicity and Health Unit at the University of Central Lancashire.

After extensive piloting of the proforma, and a training programme, Commissioners and Secretariat staff (hereafter referred to as Visitors) conducted the visits, mostly in pairs, to a sample of inpatient units for people aged primarily between 16 and 65 in England and Wales on 11 May 1999.

Units to be visited

- All 66 local authorities in England and Wales which had on or above the national average of 5.3% of their population from black and minority ethnic communities, or had at least 10,000 residents from these groups, were identified. One NHS acute mental health unit in each area was randomly selected to be visited.

- Sixteen units for people with learning disabilities, which had at least one detained patient from black and minority ethnic communities, were selected randomly.

- Sixteen NHS medium secure units were selected randomly from those which had at least three detained patients from black and minority ethnic communities.

- Eight independent sector medium secure units were selected randomly from those which had at least three detained patients from black and minority ethnic communities.

- Four independent sector acute units were selected randomly from those which had at least three detained patients from black and minority ethnic communities.

- All three of the NHS high secure hospitals were selected.

Some units were withdrawn from the sample when they were found not to meet the agreed criteria, and not all the planned visits took place due to unavoidable circumstances on the day.

Advance Notification

The Commission formally notified, some time in advance, all units providing care for detained patients in England and Wales that it would be undertaking a Second National Visit. It specified the four issues relating to patients from black and minority ethnic groups which were to be considered, and informed the units that some of them would be included in the Visit. Selected units received about two weeks notice of the date of the visit.

The Visit

The Visit comprised three parts:

SECTION A: An announced visit to the Unit General Manager

Based on the previous work by the Commission, already detailed, four specific issues were chosen for attention, and the unit managers had been asked to have available for inspection all written policies, procedures or guidelines on these issues. Visitors collected copies of many of these for further examination, in order to identify examples of good practice. Managers were asked about their services' policies, and their practice, on:

- **recording the ethnicity of patients (with supplementary questions about what use they made of this information);**

- **dealing with racial harassment of black and minority ethnic patients by other patients, or by staff;**

- **training in race equality and anti-discriminatory practice for staff;**

- **provision of, access to and use of interpreters.**

Additional questions about the care provided for black and minority ethnic patients elicited information on other examples of good practice, for example in the provision of information packs on different cultural and religious groups, their customs and festivals.

Policies shown to the Visitors which were labelled 'Draft', and those dated May 1999, were excluded, as were Action Plans which lacked any indication of how they would be implemented and monitored.

The presence of written policies on the various issues cannot be taken as proof of good practice, nor does their absence necessarily denote poor practice. However, having a policy indicates an issue has at least been considered, and is a more reliable way of guiding practice than word of mouth or custom and practice. Visitors followed up questions on policies with an exploration of practice at unit, ward and patient levels, to determine to what extent they were being followed.

S E C T I O N   B :   An unannounced visit to a randomly selected ward

Following the interview with the Unit Manager, Visitors asked to interview the manager of a ward selected at random from all those which currently had detained black and minority ethnic patients. This part of the visit had **not** been announced in advance. Ward managers were asked about policies and practice relating to the same issues as had been covered with the Unit Managers.

S E C T I O N   C :   An examination of patients' notes

After interviewing the ward managers, Visitors asked to see the case notes of a number of black and minority ethnic detained patients; these were selected according to a system designed to eliminate bias. Visitors established what information was recorded on each patient relating to age, gender, ethnicity, religion, language and dialect. They also asked how individuals' religious and cultural needs had been taken into account in the care provided.

Table 1 shows the number of units and wards visited in each category, and the number of patients whose notes were examined.

Table 1 *Number of units and wards visited, and number of case notes of black and minority ethnic detained patients examined, by type of unit*

	Acute	Learning Disabilities	NHS Secure	Independent Secure	Independent Acute	NHS High Secure	**Total**
Units	61	14	14	8	4	3	**104**
Wards	61	14	14	8	4	18	**119**
Patients	343	30	52	36	14	59	**534**

Altogether data was obtained on 534 patients from black and minority ethnic groups who were detained on 11 May 1999.

The sample for National Visit 2 was deliberately constructed to focus on areas of the country where there are significant black and minority ethnic communities. The results published in this report are therefore highly relevant to all inpatient units who need to meet the needs of people from these communities. However, because the sample was focused and not random, it is not possible to estimate from these figures the proportion of detained patients in the whole of England and Wales who come from black and minority ethnic groups.

This preliminary report presents some of the findings from this the Second National Visit, in which an enormous amount of data was collected.

In each of the following sections, we present major findings from the quantitative data, and some examples of good practice, followed by a discussion. Where it aids clarity, we include verbatim the questions asked by the Visitors.

This report will not attempt to compare responses between the different types of units and wards visited; information will be presented as a whole, for example across all units, all wards, or for all patients.

Some examples of current good practice on ethnic monitoring, dealing with racial harassment, training in race equality and anti-discriminatory practice for staff and the provision, access to and use of interpreters, are included, with contact details for those organisations provided.

Further detailed work on the quantitative data, and analysis of the qualitative data, is yet to take place. In addition, we have received a great deal of information on good practice, which contributes to the care and treatment of black and minority ethnic patients, but which falls outside the specific categories listed above; this is yet to be analysed.

There will be further dissemination of our findings later this year, including articles in professional, managerial and academic journals, and will include practical advice on improving care for black and minority ethnic patients through a series of good practice checklists.

RECORDING ETHNICITY AND OTHER DEMOGRAPHIC DATA ON DETAINED PATIENTS

Introduction

Since 1995, NHS Trusts have been required to record the ethnicity of all patients admitted; this is also mandatory for independent sector units providing care to NHS-funded inpatients.[2] Quantifying the population is only the first step in addressing the needs of patients from different ethnic groups, but it is a crucial one, and the information can be used in many ways to monitor the provision of existing services and to plan and develop future ones.

The NHS Executive Guidance on recording ethnicity (1994)[3] states: *'An ethnic group is a group of people who share characteristics such as language, history, culture, upbringing, religion, nationality, geographical and ancestral origins and place. This provides the group with a distinct identity as seen by themselves and others.'*

As this National Visit focused on the care of detained patients who are not white, the ONS classification (formerly OPCS) of ethnic groups from the 1991 Census, which is routinely used by the Commission, was used, excluding only the 'white' category. The following groups were therefore *included:*

- **Black Caribbean**
- **Black Other**
- **Pakistani**
- **Chinese**

- **Black African**
- **Indian**
- **Bangladeshi**
- **Other**

Findings

ETHNICITY

Details were obtained of the recorded ethnicity of 534 black and minority ethnic detained patients across all the units visited. Information collected on a further 60 patients was excluded from the analysis as eight of these were recorded as being white, and the other 52 had no information recorded on their ethnicity.

The biggest minority ethnic group was Black Caribbean, comprising 42% of those for whom ethnicity was recorded, with Black African and Black Other making up the next largest groups. Figure 1 shows this.

Figure 1 *Recorded ethnicity of detained black and minority ethnic patients (%)*

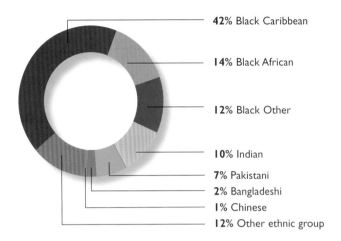

42% Black Caribbean

14% Black African

12% Black Other

10% Indian

7% Pakistani

2% Bangladeshi

1% Chinese

12% Other ethnic group

GENDER AND AGE

Information on gender was recorded for 525 of the 534 patients. Three hundred and seventy three (71%) were male and 152 (29%) were female. The age of the detained patients from black and minority ethnic groups is shown in figure 2.

Figure 2 *Age of detained patients from black and minority ethnic groups (%)*

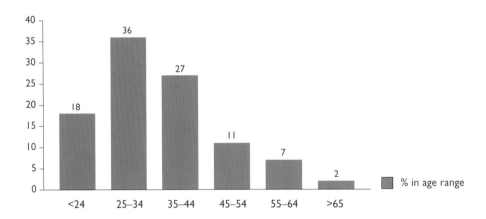

FIRST LANGUAGE, DIALECT SPOKEN, AND FLUENCY IN ENGLISH

| Question: | *What is this patient's first language? What is their second language? What dialect does this patient speak?* |

Four hundred and eighteen patients (78%) were reported to have English as their first language, with a further 72 (13%) said to speak it as a second language.

For the 116 patients whose first language was not English, the recording of their first language in their case notes, or knowledge of it by ward staff, was generally poor. These 116 patients between them spoke 26 different languages. Few examples were found of any dialect spoken; table 2 shows that language, dialect and country of origin were sometimes confused.

Table 2 *Languages spoken by the 116 black and minority ethnic detained patients whose first language was not English (NB Inverted commas indicates this is **not** a language)*

1st Language:	number	1st Language:	number
Punjabi	18	Vietnamese	1
Gujarati	10	Chinese	4
Urdu	5	Cantonese	4
Hindi	2	'Philipino'	1
'Indian'	1	Yoruba	2
Bengali	5	'Nigerian'	1
'Bangladeshi'	4	'Ghanaian'	3
Tamil	1	'Uganda'	1
Arabic	3	French	2
Somali	8	Italian	1
'Iranian'	1	Spanish	1
Kurdish	1	Makaton (sign language)	1
Turkish	2	Not given	32
Thai	1		
Total 116			

Dialects spoken by patients whose first language is not English

(NB Many of these are languages, not dialects; inverted commas indicates this is neither a language nor a dialect)

1st Language:	number	1st Language:	number
Punjabi	3	'Somalian'	1
'Philipino dialect (unspecified)'	1	Hindi/Punjabi	1
Arabic	1	Cantonese	2
Benagli	1	'Algerian Arabic'	1
'Bangladeshi'	1	'Cypriot'	1

Dialects spoken by patients whose first language is English

1st Language:	number	1st Language:	number
Patois	9	Creole	2

> **Question:** *Does this patient speak English fluently?*

Ward managers reported that four hundred and sixty nine people (88%) were fluent in English, and 56 (10%) were said to speak no English, or only a little; these 56 people could be assumed to need an interpreter during their stay in hospital. In nine cases (2%) it was not known whether or not the patient could speak English fluently. (Figure 3)

Figure 3 *Per cent of black and minority ethnic detained patients fluent in English*

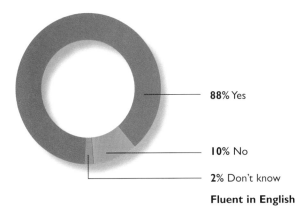

88% Yes

10% No

2% Don't know

Fluent in English

FLUENCY IN ENGLISH AND ETHNICITY

Figure 4 shows the relationship between fluency in English and ethnicity. Fluency in English ranged from 98% of Black Caribbean patients to only 50% of Bangladeshi patients.

Figure 4 *Per cent of each ethnic group who were fluent in English (%)*

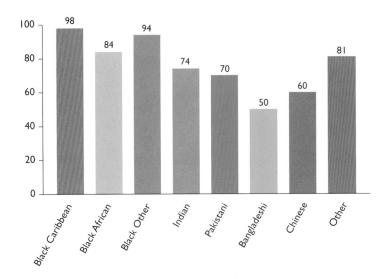

RELIGION

| Question: | *What is this patient's religion? Please also record religious sect.* |

The most commonly recorded religion was some form of Christianity (including Church of England, Roman Catholicism, Baptist, Methodist, Pentecostal, and Orthodox churches), with 189 patients comprising 35% of the total. Muslims made up the next largest group, with 103 people (19%). Information was not recorded for 46 people (9%). Other than for Christianity, religious sects were not recorded.

Figure 5 *Religion of black and minority ethnic detained patients*

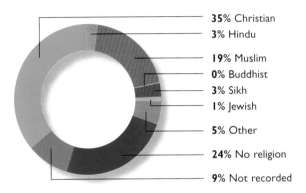

- **35**% Christian
- **3**% Hindu
- **19**% Muslim
- **0**% Buddhist
- **3**% Sikh
- **1**% Jewish
- **5**% Other
- **24**% No religion
- **9**% Not recorded

Aggregating Black Caribbean, Black African and Black Other as 'black', this group is predominately Christian. 'Asian' patients, comprising Indians, Pakistanis and Bengalis, are mostly Muslim. 'All other religions' have been aggregated for clarity; however, a significant number of Indian patients are Hindu or Sikh. The relationship between aggregated ethnic groups and the largest religious groups is shown in figure 6.

Figure 6 *Distribution of the most commonly recorded religions across aggregated ethnic groups for black and minority ethnic detained patients – number*

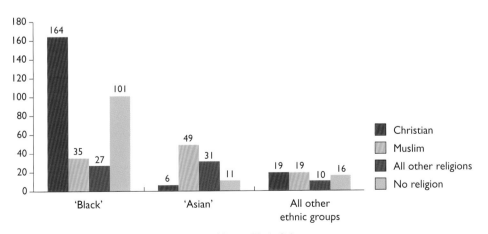

NB. **'Black'** includes: Black Caribbean, Black African, Black Other;
  'Asian' includes: Indian, Pakistani, Bangladeshi;
  'All other ethnic groups' includes: Chinese, other.

Data on patients whose religion was not recorded, or was recorded as 'don't know', have been omitted from this figure.

Discussion

In order to draw up a package of care which takes account of a patient's ethnic, cultural and communication needs, it is necessary to accurately collect and clearly record information on these issues. Although this information was present for most patients, information on ethnicity, fluency in English and religion was missing in around nine per cent of the case notes examined, and little information was recorded on dialects spoken, or religious sects. Some of what were reported to be languages and dialects are not, in fact, languages or dialects.

The lack of information on dialect spoken has significant implications for planning a care package. For example, there are two main dialects of Punjabi, Gurmukhi Punjabi generally being spoken by people of Indian origin who are Sikhs, while Mirpuri Punjabi is commonly spoken by people from Pakistan who are Muslims. Similarly, there are differences between the two dialects of Bengali. A later section of this report deals with access to and use of interpreters, but it is relevant to stress here that without knowing the language and dialect spoken by their patients, ward staff will be unable to obtain an appropriate interpreter. This interrelationship between language, dialect and religion demonstrates the importance of recording full information on all of these.

Additionally, although people from black and minority ethnic groups may be fluent in English, it should be recognised that at times of stress, including periods of mental illness, some may prefer to use their mother tongue; again, in this situation, an interpreter would be necessary, and their second language and dialect should be recorded to facilitate this.

The great diversity of languages spoken by patients will clearly present difficulties for staff trying to find appropriate interpreters in an area where there may be few people locally who speak all the relevant languages. However, without appropriate means of communication, it will be almost impossible to plan and deliver patients' care.

Further analysis of the data will examine the relationship between the age of the patients, their ethnicity and their fluency in English.

Examples of good practice in the recording and monitoring of patients' ethnicity will be presented in the next section.

Introduction

Ethnic monitoring is no more than a statistical exercise that by itself can achieve nothing. However, it is an essential tool to 'root out' discrimination, which is often covert and unintentional. Without ethnic monitoring, it is difficult to establish the nature and extent of inequality, the areas where action is most needed, and whether measures aimed at reducing inequality are succeeding.

The purpose of ethnic monitoring is extensive and can include the following:

- **determine current use of services**

- **identify gaps in the service**

- **assess health needs of the minority ethnic community**

- **improve quality of services**

- **evaluate changes in services**

- **achieve equal access to services**

- **provide a baseline for planning**

- **measure health improvements.**

Ethnic monitoring has considerable advantages. It can provide a more accurate picture of current services used by people from various communities than is otherwise available. In addition, it can raise questions about particular issues warranting further examination and they can provide a baseline for planning, target setting, and measuring change, and ultimately measuring health outcomes.

Findings – Units

Question: *Do you routinely record the ethnicity of patients on admission?*

Of the 104 units visited, 52 (50%) had a written policy on recording the ethnicity of their patients; 33 (32%) showed Visitors a written policy, with another 19 (18%) reporting they had one. Although half the units had no policy, all said they did routinely record some information on ethnicity at the time of admission, although not all used the ONS categories for this.

Figure 7 *Percentage of units with a policy on recording patients' ethnicity*

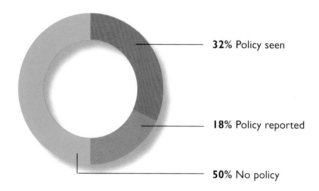

— **32%** Policy seen

— **18%** Policy reported

— **50%** No policy

Question: *Where is this information held?*

In most cases (91%), information on patients' ethnicity was held at ward level, with it being held centrally, for example at Trust level, in 81% of cases. This information was held at unit level in only 67% of cases. In most cases, the information was held in more than one location.

Figure 8 *Where data on ethnicity was held within organisations (%)*

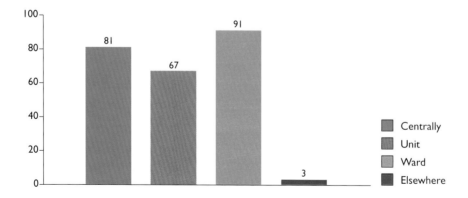

Question: *As a manager, are you required to make any returns on the ethnicity of detained patients to your central office?*

Fifty-seven of the unit managers (56%) said they were required to make regular returns on ethnicity, most to a central office, or to the Trust or independent sector provider Board. As managers in some units made returns to more than one part of their organisation, Figure 9 shows the numbers of managers making returns to each.

Figure 9 *Number of units required to make returns on patients' ethnicity, and where the information goes*

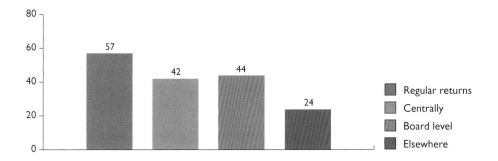

Question: *Do you use these returns to identify gaps in existing services? Do you use these returns in service planning and development?*

Thirty-six managers (35%) said the information was used to identify gaps in existing services, and 47 managers (45%) reported it being used in service planning and development. Fifty-four of the units (52%) had an officer with lead responsibility for reporting on ethnicity to the Board.

Question: *As a manager, do you use information on the ethnicity of detained patients to monitor the following:*

- **the number of compulsory admissions;**

- **use of therapies and activities;**

- **use of the Mental Health Act;**

- **self-harm;**

- **violent incidents;**

- **deaths;**

- **complaints;**

- **applications to and outcomes of Mental Health Review Tribunals;**

- **employment policies to ensure the staff employed reflect the composition of the patient population.**

Fourteen units (13%) did nothing beyond recording patients' ethnicity. The uses to which the other 90 units put it are given in figure 10; only in relation to staff employment did more than half the units make use of ethnicity data.

Figure 10 *Use made of patients' ethnicity data by units (%)*

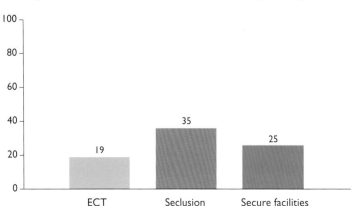

Legend:
- Compulsory admission
- Therapy
- Use of Mental Health Act
- Self harm
- Violent incidents
- Deaths
- Complaints
- Mental Health Review Tribunals
- Staff

Values: 43, 25, 48, 14, 21, 27, 27, 13, 64

| Question: | *As a manager, do you use information on the ethnicity of detained patients to monitor the following:* |

- **use of electroconvulsive therapy (ECT)**

- **use of seclusion**

- **use of secure facilities.**

These questions were not applicable to all units visited, as not all used ECT in inpatient care, some did not use seclusion, while other units entirely comprised secure provision. Altogether, ECT was given on 77 units, of which 15 (19%) used ethnicity information to monitor this; 23 (35%) of the 66 units which used seclusion monitored the ethnicity of secluded patients; and of the 71 units using secure facilities 18 of them (25%) used it to monitor the use of secure facilities. In figure 11, the units using information on ethnicity for each of these purposes is given as a percentage of these numbers.

Figure 11 *Other uses made of patients' ethnicity data by units (%)*

ECT 19
Seclusion 35
Secure facilities 25

Good practice in recording and monitoring ethnicity

From the 25 written policies obtained from the units by the Visitors there were several examples of good practice, both in recording ethnic data and in using it to monitor the delivery of the service to black and minority ethnic patients.

Wolverhampton Health Care NHS Trust has produced leaflets for patients and for staff, setting out the reasons for collecting the information and the use that will be made of it, including assurances of confidentiality and the rights of an individual to refuse. A laminated card showing the ONS categories, on which the patient can indicate their ethnicity, is written in the most common languages encountered locally.

Similarly, Thames Gateway NHS Trust (formerly North Kent Healthcare NHS Trust) has a laminated booklet designed for staff to explain ethnic monitoring, and to establish patients' ethnic group, to those speaking Bengali, Chinese, Gujarati, Hindi, Punjabi, Turkish and Urdu.

In addition to recording the ONS categories, some units have devised a secondary level of categorisation specifically to meet the diversity of their local minority ethnic communities. For example, the former West London Healthcare NHS Trust (now part of Ealing, Hammersmith & Fulham Mental Health NHS Trust), has an additional list of ethnic groups designed to assess sub-groups, based on their knowledge of the local population, including Irish, Portuguese, Turkish Cypriot, East African, Indo-Caribbean, African Asian and Vietnamese.

Some units were able to demonstrate the use they had made of ethnic monitoring data. Oxleas NHS Trust's Quarterly Information Report, January-December 1998, gives a breakdown by ethnicity of: all admissions, and readmissions within 90 days, to the acute units; complaints relating to hospital and community-based services; and the use of each of the sections of the Mental Health Act. It also assesses, and is setting further targets for, the levels of 'coding completeness', to ensure the accuracy of the data. In addition, the Trust's secure unit provides an analysis of admissions, incidents involving drugs or alcohol, and episodes of seclusion.

South Buckinghamshire NHS Trust provides some valuable guidance and information for front-line reception, admission and clerical staff with respect to a range of issues on ethnic group data collection.

Discussion

The recording of ethnicity is near to complete, with a few exceptions, but it seems the data is not being put to great use. This is disappointing, given the effort to collect data and the evidence that black and minority ethnic patients may be over-represented in terms of compulsory admissions.[4] In addition to the treatments offered to black African Caribbean people being more likely to be compulsory, they also appear to be more physical, for example drugs and ECT, instead of the more socially valued psychotherapies.[5] A small minority of wards (9%) did not keep ethnicity data on the ward, which may make the provision of a culturally sensitive service to individual patients almost impossible. It is interesting to note that more units used ethnicity information for staffing purposes (64%) than for any direct patient-related purpose.

DEALING WITH RACIAL HARASSMENT OF BLACK AND MINORITY ETHNIC PATIENTS BY OTHER PATIENTS, OR BY STAFF

Introduction

Racial harassment is an offensive and unacceptable, but not uncommon, experience in the everyday lives of people from black and minority ethnic groups. Racial harassment not only includes physical attacks on individuals but also verbal abuse and other forms of behaviour that deter people from using or participating in a particular service. Racial harassment can be deliberate and conscious, but it can also be unintentional such as banter which is insensitive to another person's feelings, and is racially or culturally offensive.

The Department of Health has drawn up a plan to end racial harassment in the NHS by embarking on a zero tolerance campaign which would challenge racial harassment of both staff and patients with perpetrators facing the threat of prosecution (Dept. of Health 1999).[6]

In the previous National Visit, we found 34 of the 291 mixed wards visited (12%) had policies on preventing and dealing with the harassment of women patients.[7] This time we looked at how units and the wards dealt with the racial harassment of patients by other patients, or by staff.

Findings – Units

> **Question:** *Are there any written policies, procedures or guidelines on dealing with the racial harassment of black and minority ethnic patients by other patients?*

Seventy-six units (73%) had no written policy on dealing with racial harassment of patients by other patients. Nineteen units (18%) showed Visitors such a policy, and a further 9 (9%) reported having one although did not produce it.

> **Question:** *Are there any written policies, procedures or guidelines on dealing with the racial harassment of black and minority ethnic patients by staff?*

Similarly, 75 units (72%) had no policy on dealing with racial harassment by staff. Nineteen unit policies (18%) were seen, and a further 10 units (10%) were reported to have one. More units than this initially reported having such a policy, but on examination many of these were found to relate to racial harassment of staff at work, and to equal opportunities in employment. Although no doubt good practice, these were outside the scope of the visit and were therefore excluded.

Figure 12 *Percentage of units with policies on racial harassment of black and minority ethnic patients*

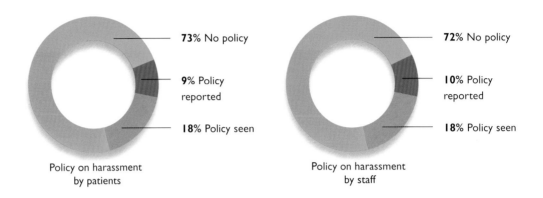

73% No policy	**72**% No policy
9% Policy reported	**10**% Policy reported
18% Policy seen	**18**% Policy seen

Policy on harassment by patients　　　　Policy on harassment by staff

Question: *Whether or not there is a written policy on this, how do you deal with incidents of racial harassment of black and minority ethnic patients on your Unit – by other patients or by staff? Please give examples of your success in this area, and/or say what the obstacles are to dealing effectively with it.*

Despite the lack of a written policy in many cases, 81 unit managers (78%) were able to describe steps they were taking to deal with racial harassment of patients by other patients, and 76 (73%) could describe what they would do in the case of racial harassment of patients by staff. However, half the units reported having difficulties in dealing with racial harassment of patients by other patients, while a third reported problems in dealing with racial harassment of patients by staff. This data will be further analysed later.

Findings – Wards

Question: *Are there any written policies, procedures or guidelines on dealing with the racial harassment of black and minority ethnic patients by other patients? If so, are the staff aware of it; how do you know? If so, are the patients aware of it; how do you know?*

Seventy-nine ward managers (66%) said they had no policy on dealing with racial harassment of patients by patients which was kept on the ward, and 24 (20%) did not know if there was one.

Sixteen managers (13%) said they had such a policy. Of these, 12 managers thought the staff on their ward knew about the policy, and six thought the patients were aware of it.

Question: *Are there any written policies, procedures or guidelines on dealing with the racial harassment of black and minority ethnic patients by staff? If so, are the staff aware of it; how do you know? If so, are the patients aware of it; how do you know?*

Similarly, 72 wards (61%) had no policy on dealing with racial harassment of patients by staff, and 26 (22%) did not know if there was one. On the 21 wards (17%) which reported having such a policy, 17 managers thought their staff knew of the policy, and eight thought the patients were aware of it.

Figure 13 *Number of wards with policies on racial harassment of patients, and the awareness of staff and patients about the policy*

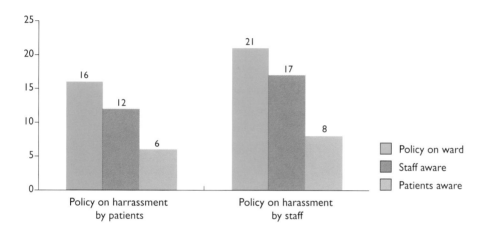

Question: *Have there been any incidents of racial harassment of black and minority ethnic patients, during the last 6 months? This includes racial harassment by other patients, or by staff.*

Twenty nine wards (24%) described an incident of racial harassment of a patient, during the last six months, which had been successfully dealt with, while ten (8%) described one which had been less successfully handled.

Findings – Patients

Question: *Has this patient ever complained of being racially harassed on this ward? If yes, please say what happened and how it was dealt with.*

Ward staff were asked whether the patients whose notes had been selected for examination had ever complained of being racially harassed; this had been the case for 59 patients (11%).

Good practice in dealing with racial harassment of patients

Only five written policies on dealing with the racial harassment of patients were obtained by Visitors. Despite this overall lack, there were some striking examples of services which were taking this issue very seriously, and had produced documents to guide staff in ensuring racial harassment was not tolerated.

South Buckinghamshire NHS Trust's Policy on the Protection of Vulnerable Adults includes racial harassment in the category of 'psychological abuse', which denies an individual's basic human and civil rights, for example with regard to following spiritual or cultural beliefs, and including racial abuse and harassment. It also details examples of 'institutional abuse' such as the lack of choice regarding diet and menus, and ignoring patients' religious needs. After listing some signs to alert staff to possible abuse, a clear procedure is set out, making the point that this is the same whether the alleged abuser is another patient, a member of staff or a visitor. The policy also details communication, religious, dietary and other issues that should be taken into account when dealing with the protection of vulnerable adults.

The former Pathfinder Mental Health Services NHS Trust (now South West London and St George's Mental Health NHS Trust) has a Racial Harassment Procedure as part of its anti-racist strategy, aiming to make it easier for people to report racial harassment and covering aspects of prevention and action to be taken. It starts from the premise that, as part of its work towards improving mental health it must 'confront discrimination and racism, whether direct or indirect, and promote equal access and anti-racist practice in all aspects of policies and practice'. It includes measures both to protect and support the person who is experiencing harassment, and to deal with the perpetrator, and is linked with the Trust's ongoing staff training programme, which is mandatory for all new and existing staff. The policy states that complaints of racial harassment must always be treated 'seriously, sensitively and promptly', and must be fully investigated and documented, using the same procedure for complaints about patients or staff. There is also a commitment to keeping under review the level and type of complaints of racial harassment, and acting on the findings.

The Spinney in Manchester has adopted a policy on harassment and equal opportunities in service provision which reflect the King's Fund Organisational Audit Standard. This provides a clear statement that reports of racial harassment will be taken very seriously and dealt with sympathetically and quickly. It aims to encourage the victim to come forward and, recognising the sensitive personal nature of many complaints of harassment, it also provides for some choice as to whom the complaint can be made. Quarterly monitoring information is provided to the senior management team for appropriate action.

Discussion

We were disappointed to see so few policies on dealing with racial harassment on the wards, which was similar to our previous findings on dealing with the sexual harassment of women. However, the quality of the few policies which were presented to Visitors was high.

Finding 59 recorded instances of racial harassment among the patients whose notes were selected, representing 11% of the total, is of great concern, given the number of filters operating – i.e. an incident has to be reported to staff, acknowledged as racial harassment, and recorded in the case notes. Further analysis will show whether these incidents occurred across all types of unit visited, or whether they were more common in some types of services than in others, and may also shed light on the nature of the obstacles to progress in addressing staff training needs.

One possible way of dealing with racial harassment by another patient is to move the harasser from the ward. During several of the pilot visits, we found examples of the *victims* of racial harassment being moved from the wards, either because other wards were reluctant to take the perpetrators, or for clinical reasons. There is a danger that the victim of racial harassment can thus be doubly disadvantaged.

As the good practice examples show, it is important to note that racial harassment is not only something which is 'done to' patients in the form of verbal or physical abuse, but it is also about the non-provision of appropriate services for black and minority ethnic groups. This will be covered further in subsequent dissemination.

TRAINING IN RACE EQUALITY AND ANTI-DISCRIMINATORY PRACTICE FOR STAFF, AND THE PROVISION OF CULTURALLY-SENSITIVE CARE

Introduction

It is a requirement of the Patient's Charter that health services respect an individual's privacy, dignity, and cultural and religious beliefs. In order to provide mental health care which is sensitive to the needs of all its patients, staff need appropriate training and information to equip them for this role. We live in an increasingly multi-cultural environment, in which 5.3% of the overall population of England and Wales belong to black and minority ethnic groups. Staff in areas where these communities are relatively small may feel under-prepared to deal with patients from these groups or, having recognised their training needs, may be particularly sensitised and well-prepared for the issues. Paradoxically, those in more ethnically mixed areas may be more complacent and less aware, through habituation.

Providing training for all staff is a positive step, as is the development of a policy on race equality and anti-discriminatory practice. However, we should also remember that patients should still be able to exercise individual choice, and that not everyone conforms to strict religious or cultural norms.

Findings – Units

Question: *Are there any written policies, procedures or guidelines on training in race equality and anti-discriminatory practice for staff?*

Seventy units (67%) had no policy on this. Twenty-three (22%) unit policies were seen, and a further 11 (11%) were reported.

Figure 14 *Percentage of units with policies on training for staff in race equality and anti-discriminatory practice*

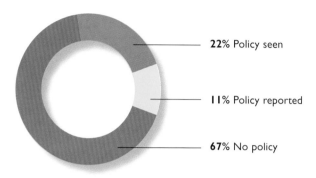

22% Policy seen

11% Policy reported

67% No policy

Question: *Do all your staff receive training in race equality and anti-discriminatory practice? If so, is this training requirement included in staffs' job descriptions?*

Seventy-one units (68%) did not provide training for all staff in anti-discriminatory practice. In 75 units (84%) there was no requirement for staff to undergo such training, although this was a requirement which was included in job descriptions in 11 units (12%).

Findings – Patients

Question: *Have any specific therapeutic activities been undertaken that reflect the ethnicity and culture of this patient? Are there any specific recreational activities available on this ward which reflect their ethnicity and culture?*

Ward staff reported that for 355 (67%) and 354 (67%) patients respectively, there had been no specific therapeutic or recreational activities that reflected the patients' ethnicity, religion and culture.

Figure 15 *Per cent of black and minority ethnic detained patients who received therapeutic and recreational activities which reflected their ethnicity and culture*

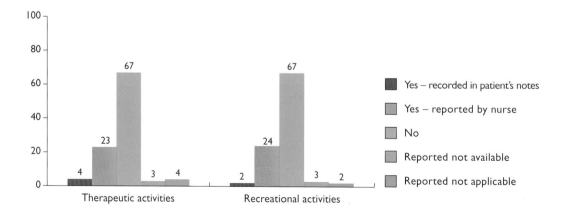

Good practice in training in race equality and anti-discriminatory practice for staff, and the provision of culturally-sensitive care

Information was obtained from twenty-eight units on programmes of training for staff. However, few of these programmes dealt directly with race equality and anti-discriminatory practice, and most were aimed at improving staffs' understanding of a range of religious and cultural issues in respect of patient care, in many cases supplemented by information packs, held at ward level, providing guidance on cultural and religious practices. Several of these, as well as appearing to be very well researched and comprehensive in their coverage, were attractively presented and easily accessible to staff seeking guidance. Many included calendars showing the dates of the festivals for all major religions in the current year.

Guild Community Health Care NHS Trust has been running black and minority ethnic cultural awareness training twice yearly since 1995, open to all Trust staff, and comprising workshops and seminar presentations. Local evaluation has shown staff find the course informative and interesting.

Wolverhampton Health Care NHS Trust's inter-cultural awareness training resource includes useful sections on naming systems, languages, religion and customs of a number of minority ethnic groups, whilst clearly making the point that generalisation about the cultural, social and religious backgrounds of minority ethnic groups can be very misleading.

North Manchester Healthcare NHS Trust runs a course on Muslim cultural awareness, including much background information on the faith, its customs and requirements, and a local Islamic organisation in Manchester has organised a seminar for Trust staff on caring for Muslims in hospital.

Broadmoor Hospital Authority's programme of continuing professional development includes sessions entitled 'Working with Difference' which aims to enable staff to reflect on their practice and to facilitate new ways of working with differences and diversity. The programme consists of weekly sessions over ten weeks, plus directed study time, a clinical placement day and a review day. Five modules cover: towards an understanding of transcultural issues; analysing power; service delivery and practice issues in caring for black patients; towards better service provision for mentally ill people from ethnic minorities; evaluating service delivery – the challenge. The hospital has also run programmes of events for 'Africa Week' and 'Multi Cultural Week', comprising talks, discussions, food demonstration and tasting, music and dancing.

As part of the work of the Race and Culture Group at Broadmoor Hospital, standards covering anti-discriminatory training, diet, personal care, and religious and spiritual needs have been drawn up, and an audit carried out with staff and patients to assess their successful implementation. Although this showed less than universal understanding of race and cultural issues at ward level, it has provided managers with a benchmark against which they can monitor future progress, and an action plan, with clearly identified milestones, for the next steps to be taken.

BHB Community Health Care NHS Trust has a comprehensive information pack for staff on ethnic and religious minority groups, produced by the local user group, HUBB (Havering Users Barking and Brentwood). The format of a ring-binder with inserts makes it easy to add to, or update, the information. It also includes addresses of various local organisations who may be a useful contact for staff or patients, and a list of key personnel in the Trust who have responsibility for some aspect of service provision for minority ethnic communities.

Northwest Anglia Healthcare NHS Trust, Northampton Community Healthcare NHS Trust, Broadmoor Hospital Authority, North Warwickshire NHS Trust, Community Health Care Service North Derbyshire NHS Trust, St Andrew's Hospital in Northampton, and Kneesworth House Psychiatric Hospital all have comprehensive information packs. However, not all units have compiled their own information packs, nor is it necessary always to start from scratch. In addition to its own quick reference guide to cultural awareness – one sheet of laminated card which provides a good starting point – Dudley Priority Health NHS Trust makes use of more detailed materials on religious festivals compiled by the Shap Working Party on World Religions in Education, a registered educational charity. Another Trust makes use of a cultural awareness guide produced by Portsmouth Healthcare NHS Trust.

Discussion

Although there were some signs that staffs' training needs in race equality and anti-discriminatory practice were beginning to be addressed, this was happening in only a minority of units. This will be particularly important for the units in this survey, which were selected because of the ethnic diversity of their catchment areas. It should also be acknowledged that there is a considerable training agenda for mental health staff in many areas of their work.[8,9] However, good practice will only become ingrained when all units have policies which are fully implemented so that staff have received training.

8 | PROVISION OF, ACCESS TO, AND USE OF INTERPRETERS

Introduction

The issue of the availability, training and use of interpreters has been a long-standing area of concern for the MHAC, whose routine visit reports have continued to suggest that this area remains a low priority for service providers.[10] The areas of concern range from: a lack of staff training in the use of interpreters, the bad practice of using cleaning staff, relatives and even other patients as interpreters, through to the unavailability of trained and qualified interpreters. When interpreters have been available they have not always appeared to be used appropriately, for example, interpreters' availability does not always coincide with ward rounds or when the patient needs them most. These and many other issues can lead to patients' rights not being adequately explained to them, and very little therapeutic help provided, leaving them even more isolated and anxious.

It is always preferable for patients to communicate to a mental health professional who can understand their culture and language, and providers should seek to recruit staff from relevant backgrounds. However, there is likely to be a continuing need for interpreters, who should be given training not only in interpreting but also in mental health situations; similarly, staff should be trained in the use of interpreters.

The principle of ensuring effective communication with the patient is enshrined in Section 13(2) of the Mental Health Act (1983):

'Before making an application for the admission of a patient to hospital an approved social worker shall interview the patient in a suitable manner...'

Prominence is given to issues of communication in the first chapter of the revised Code of Practice,[11] where it is stated:

'Local and Health Authorities and Trusts should ensure that ASWs, doctors, nurses and others receive sufficient guidance in the use of interpreters and should make arrangements for there to be an easily accessible pool of trained interpreters. Authorities and Trusts should consider co-operating in making this provision' (1.4)

The MHAC in its very first Biennial Report (1985)[12] identified several practical measures that needed to be introduced, including:

- **Centrally translated leaflets in appropriate languages should be made available for those whose first language is not English and tape recordings made for those who have difficulty in reading and writing any language.**

- **That an effective joint health and social services interpreting service should be established. It is inappropriate to rely on family members, particularly children, or other bilingual members of staff. This would ensure information is available to patients and relatives both before admission and during a patient's stay.**

Seven Biennial Reports later, these common-sense suggestions have not yet been fully implemented.

Findings – Units

Question: *Are there any written policies, procedures or guidelines on the provision and use of interpreters?*

Fifty-two units (50%) had a policy on the provision and use of interpreters.

Figure 16 *Units with policies on provision of, access to, and use of interpreters (%)*

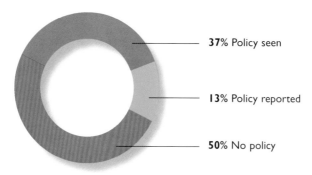

37% Policy seen

13% Policy reported

50% No policy

Question: *How has your Unit dealt with the issue of providing and using interpreters? Have you ever used an independent interpreter in this Unit? (i.e. either an interpreter who comes in from outside the hospital, or a member of staff who has been trained and has specific responsibility for this.)*

One hundred unit managers (96%) provided some information on positive steps they had taken to make interpreters available in their unit, although only 94 (90%) said they had ever used an independent interpreter in the unit.

Question: *Do you __ever__ use non-trained hospital staff as interpreters? Do you __ever__ use patients' relatives as interpreters?*

Sixty-one units (59%) had used non-trained staff as interpreters at some time, and 59 (57%) had used relatives. (Figure 17) Although the question demanded a 'yes' or 'no' answer, a number of units, as yet unquantified, insisted they only used non-trained staff, relatives or friends to interpret in an emergency, or to ask simple questions about, for example, dietary needs.

Figure 17 *Use of independent interpreters and non-professional interpreters by units (%)*

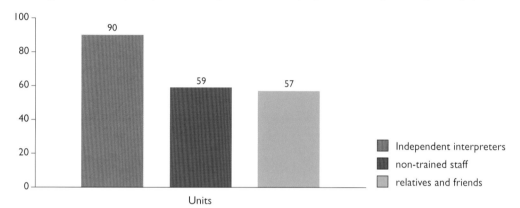

Question: *Are the interpreters trained in interpreting? Are the interpreters trained in mental health issues?*

Seventy-six units (73%) said the interpreters they used were trained in interpreting, but only 40 (39%) said they had received any form of mental health training.

Figure 18 *Units reporting on the training received by the interpreters they use (%)*

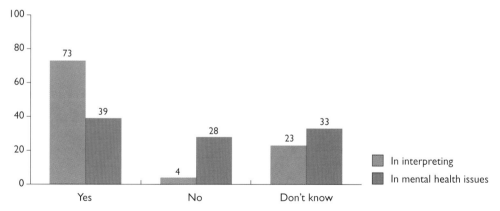

Question: **Are your staff trained in the use of interpreters?**

Seventy-four units (71%) said their staff were not trained in the use of interpreters.

Question: **Are interpreters available to all groups of staff (e.g. doctors, nurses, OTs, psychologists, advocates etc)? Are interpreters available 'out of hours'?**

Ninety-seven units (93%) reported that interpreters were available to all groups of staff, and seventy-seven (74%) said they were available in the evenings and at weekends.

Findings – wards

Fifty-nine ward managers (50%) said they had a policy on accessing and using interpreters. (Figure 19) On the 46 wards (37%) which had a policy kept either on the ward or elsewhere, 36 managers thought their staff were aware of it and 18 thought the patients were.

Figure 19 *Per cent of wards with policies on access to and use of interpreters*

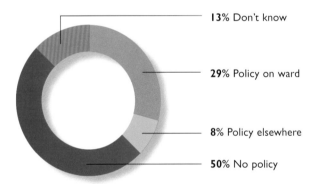

13% Don't know

29% Policy on ward

8% Policy elsewhere

50% No policy

Question: **Do you ever use patients' family members or friends to interpret for them? Do you ever use professional staff members (e.g. doctors, nurses) or non-professional staff (e.g. clerical and ancilliary staff) to interpret?**

Eighty wards (67%) had used patients' relatives or friends to interpret. Eighty-five wards (71%) had used non-trained professional staff, and 30 wards (25%) had used non-professional staff. As with the unit managers, an as yet unquantified number of ward managers insisted this was done only in an emergency, or to ask simple questions.

Question: **Have the interpreters had any training or induction on mental health issues? Are they familiar with the ward and its philosophy?**

Eighty-three of the ward managers, (70%) did not know whether the interpreters they used had received any mental health induction or training and only 18 (15%) said the interpreters were familiar with the ward and its philosophy.

Question: *Are your staff trained in the use of interpreters?*

The managers of 104 wards (87%) said their staff were not trained to use interpreters, and only ten ward managers (9%) reported this training was available to some or all of the ward staff.

Question: *In which of these ways are interpreters available: in person, on the phone?*

One hundred and ten ward managers (92%) said interpreters were available in person, and 34 (29%) could access them over the telephone.

Question: *Do the ward staff spend time with the interpreter before an interview, explaining what information is needed and why? Do they spend time with the interpreter after the interview?*

Asked about the conduct of interviews using interpreters, 82 ward managers (69%) reported that staff always or usually spent time with the interpreter before the interview. Seventy-two wards (61%) said staff always or usually spent time with the interpreter in debriefing after an interview.

Figure 20 *Wards (%) in which meetings take place with interpreters before and after interviews*

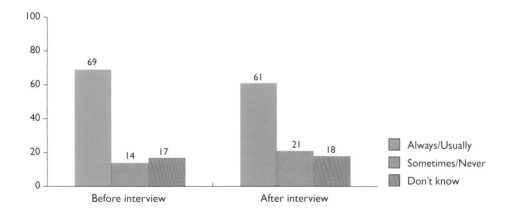

Question: *Are interpreters routinely available for nursing and medical staff? And for social work and advocacy staff?*

At the ward level, ninety-four mangers (80%) said interpreters were available to nurses and medical staff, and eighty-seven (76%) to social work and advocacy staff.

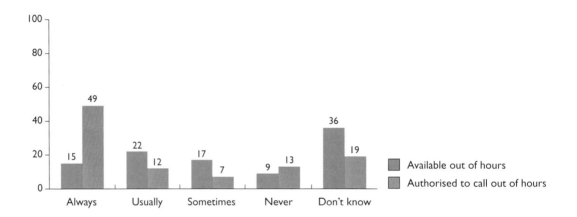

Question: *Can your staff get hold of an interpreter at night and weekends?*
Are you authorised to call an interpreter 'out of hours'?

Seventy two (61%) ward managers said they were authorised to call interpreters out of hours, for example at night and weekends, although 43 (36%) were unable to say whether they could obtain one at these times as they had never put it to the test.

Figure 21 *Wards reporting the availability of interpreters out of hours and their authorisation to call them at these times (%)*

Question: *Has an independent interpreter (i.e. an interpreter who comes in from outside the hospital, or a member of staff who has been trained and has specific responsibility for this) ever been used on this ward?*

Thirty-six (30%) of the ward managers had never used an independent interpreter on the ward. In ninety-eight cases, (82%) either a list of interpreters was accessible on the ward or elsewhere, or the arrangements were handled by an agency contact.

Findings – patients

Question: *Can patients request an interpreter?*

One hundred and four (89%) ward managers said that patients could request an interpreter, but only 36 of these could give an example of a patient having done so.

Question: *Does this patient speak fluent English? Has an interpreter ever been used with this patient?*

Fifty-six patients were not fluent in English, and it was not known whether a further nine people were fluent. Only 31 patients had ever used an interpreter.

Good practice in the use of interpreters

Twenty five units provided Visitors with policies which stated their commitment to ensuring all patients had access to someone who spoke their own language, and which explained the circumstances in which interpreters were to be used. In addition, many units had either developed their own range of written material to enable staff to have limited communication with patients who did not speak English, or were using materials compiled by other organisations.

The Code of Practice for Sessional Interpreters/Translators devised by the former West London Healthcare NHS Trust (now part of Ealing, Hammersmith and Fulham NHS Trust) states the aim of providing 'appropriate, acceptable and equitable interpreters to users, carers and professionals that are responsive to the individual needs of users and their carers from ethnic minorities'. A number of principles guide the conduct of interpreters in the implementation of the code of practice, including issues of confidentiality, impartiality and freedom from bias, and the process of an interpreted interview is spelt out in detail, to ensure the most effective outcome.

Specific guidelines to help health staff work effectively with interpreters has been produced by Lambeth, Southwark and Lewisham Health Commission Interpreting Service (used by the former West Lambeth Trust, now part of South London and Maudsley NHS Trust). These divide the interpreting process into stages of the pre-interview, introductions, client interview and post interview, explaining the purpose of each and how each should be conducted. The guidelines also include the process when the interpreter has been booked by the client, rather than the health care staff, in which case the pre-meeting is between the client and the interpreter.

The Good Practice Guidelines for the use of interpreters with patients having special communication needs produced by Rampton Hospital Authority, includes the point that although some clients may appear to speak good English, many complex issues are discussed in the context of mental health care which may be better facilitated by an interpreter to ensure good mutual understanding. The guidelines make provision for interpreters to be used for the full range of legal, therapeutic and social contacts, both one to one and in larger gatherings.

North Warwickshire NHS Trust sets out a number of problems which may arise with untrained non-professional interpreters, including a misunderstanding of their role, lack of confidentiality, bias and distortion and a lack of explanation of cultural differences. They explain the problems of using children, other family members, and friends to interpret, as well as potential difficulties with unofficial interpreters from the local community, and using non-professional and professional staff from within the health care organisation itself.

Barnet Healthcare NHS Trust's code of practice for staff using interpreting services is a short, simple and clear guide to the conduct of an interview using an interpreter.

Northampton Community Healthcare NHS Trust's Ethnic Factfile includes useful information on the languages spoken by people from different ethnic groups, including African Caribbean people who, it points out, speak English but may also speak a patois which combines elements of English, Western European and West African languages.

The Language Indicator Prompt System (Lips), developed by Haringey Council in north London, is used by several units, including Thames Gateway NHS Trust (formerly North Kent Healthcare NHS Trust). Designed as an attractive booklet, it enables staff to communicate adequately with people who can read their own language, while making arrangements for an interpreter. Key phrases, to which the worker points, include 'please take a seat while we locate an interpreter', and 'the interpreter will be here at xx time'. In addition, the Trust has devised its own set of introduction cards with which staff can communicate, including a 16 language 'pick and point' card on which patients can indicate the language spoken, and request an interpreter.

Although best practice dictates that an interpreter should be physically present to conduct an interview, there may be emergency situations in which this is not possible. In these instances, contact may be made with an interpreter over the telephone. North West Anglia Healthcare NHS Trust, in common with several others, uses Language Line, a national telephone interpreting service. Interpreters with this service are accredited with the Institute of Linguists. Their guide to good practice spells out the particular requirements of a service which is not provided face to face.

Discussion

A minority of detained patients required an interpreter during their hospital admission, and many units and wards had well-established procedures for accessing them, although there were problems in some areas where they were only infrequently required. It is worrying that not all the patients identified as not fluent in English had used an interpreter. Another concern was the widespread use of family members as interpreters which can compromise objective decision-making by staff. We will examine the descriptive accounts of the last time an interpreter was used with each individual in the next stage of data analysis.

If units are using interpreters, it is not unreasonable to expect them to know whether those staff have been trained in interpreting skills, and perhaps accredited with the Institute of Linguists. The managers' general lack of knowledge about the services they were using is worrying.

If interpreters are to provide the most effective service possible, it would be beneficial if they had had some basic induction into the mental health setting in which they were called to work, with information provided about, for example, the Mental Health Act, commonly used medication, and the nature and function of the unit in which they are being asked to work.

One immediate effect of the Visit, and of the many pilot visits which preceded it, has been to raise the awareness of managers and staff in many units to the specific issues of caring for patients from black and ethnic minorities, which is a necessary precursor to any change in practice.

Following the Visit, the Mental Health Act Commission sent a questionnaire to 80 of the NHS Trusts visited, of which 65 (80%) responded.

- Most of those who responded found the meeting with Visitors very thought provoking, and helpful in raising their awareness of how ethnic monitoring information could contribute to the management of services for detained patients.

- Most said the information discussed during the visit would help them in the future auditing of their current policies and practice, and that it would help them to develop or make changes in these policies and practice.

- Most felt that units which had not been part of the Second National Visit would find the information in the proforma a useful contribution to future planning.

- Despite these positive responses, most units said that the Commission would need to balance the benefits coming from the exercise with the inevitable burden on staff time that was a consequence of the Visit.

10 | CONCLUSION

Since its inception, the Mental Health Act Commission has been concerned about the care and treatment of patients from black and minority ethnic groups detained under the Mental Health Act. Patients from these communities may suffer additional disadvantage; environments may not be sensitive to their cultural backgrounds, and they may experience harassment. For some patients, communication with staff may be impossible unless interpreters are available. To help rectify these disadvantages, it is essential that patients' ethnicity, language and religion are recorded and monitored, and used in individual care programmes as well as in service planning and delivery.

National Visit 2 has provided a detailed assessment of the current arrangements for the care of detained people from black and minority ethnic communities:

- Information on ethnicity, language and religion was present for most patients but was sometimes obviously inaccurate, for example nationality, languages and dialects being confused with each other. Only half the units visited had clear policies on recording ethnicity.

- Most wards make use of interpreters, but still have to make inappropriate use at times of family members for communicating with patients who do not speak English.

- Information on ethnicity was used for some monitoring purposes in 87% of units; it was more common to see units using ethnicity data to monitor staffing than for direct patient-related purposes.

- Racial harassment had been identified and recorded in the notes of 11% of the patients in the sample. This no doubt under-estimates the true extent of harassment. Disappointingly, few wards could show Visitors a policy on dealing with racial harassment.

- There were some good examples of units beginning to address staff training needs in the area of race equality and anti-discriminatory practice. However, only a minority of units could show Visitors a policy on training.

On a more positive note, the Visitors were shown some excellent examples of good practice in all the areas examined. Further dissemination from National Visit 2 will share this work with the rest of the mental health field. Additionally, service providers and commissioners may want to use some of the methods used here for ongoing audit. There is good practice in the care of detained patients from black and minority ethnic communities – the challenge now is to make this common practice.

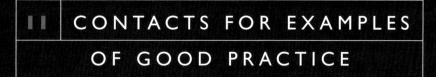

Audit and evaluation

Although the questionnaire used in the second National Visit was specifically designed as a research tool, units wanting to assess their own provision of services for black and minority ethnic groups might find the questions a useful starting point. Copies of the questionnaire can be obtained from:

The Mental Health Act Commission:
Iain Marley
The Mental Health Act Commission
Maid Marian House
56 Hounds Gate
Nottingham NG1 4QL
Telephone: 0115 943 7100

Additionally, the Sainsbury Centre is currently developing a Cultural Sensitivity Audit Tool (CAT), which is due to be published later this year. It will be available from:

The Sainsbury Centre for Mental Health:
Publications Department
The Sainsbury Centre for Mental Health
134-138 Borough High Street
London SE1 1LB
Telephone: 020 7403 8790

The units which provided Visitors with written examples of policies, procedures and guidelines in each category are listed here, along with contact details for further information. Similar details for organisations responsible for the production of other information received during the Visit are also given.

Recording and monitoring the ethnicity of patients

Ealing, Hammersmith & Fulham Mental Health NHS Trust:

Lynne Hunt
Director of Nursing
Ealing, Hammersmith & Fulham Mental Health NHS Trust
Uxbridge Road
Southall
Middlesex UB1 3EU
Telephone: 020 8354 8846

Oxleas NHS Trust:

Nick Bentley, Mental Health Act Manager
Telephone: 01322 625760

Thames Gateway NHS Trust:

Mrs Kaye Lyons, Community Liaison Manager
Telephone: 01634 234000

Mike O'Meara, Directorate Manager for Mental Health.
Telephone: 01634 380000

South Buckinghamshire NHS Trust:

Miss Jenny Cook
General Manager – Mental Health Services
South Buckinghamshire NHS Trust
Haleacre Unit
Amersham Hospital
Whielden Street
Amersham HP7 0JD
Telephone: 01494 734010

Wolverhampton Health Care NHS Trust:

Liz Richards, Mental Health Act Manager
Telephone: 01902 643149

Raj Ramkorun, Senior Nurse Co-ordinator
Telephone: 01902 643153

Wolverhampton Health Care NHS Trust
Mental Health Directorate
Wrekin House
New Cross Hospital
Wolverhampton WV10 0TT

Dealing with racial harassment of black and minority ethnic patients by other patients, or by staff

South Buckinghamshire NHS Trust:

as before

South West London and St George's Mental Health NHS Trust:

Paul Henry
Director of Human Resources
South West London and St George's Mental Health NHS Trust
Springfield University Hospital
61 Glenburnie Road
London SW17 7DJ
Telephone: 020 8682 6448

The Spinney:

Miss Margaret Gallagher
Clinical Services Manager
The Spinney
Everest Road
Atherton
Manchester M46 9NT
Telephone: 01942 88530

Training in race equality and anti-discriminatory practice for staff, and information on providing culturally sensitive care

BHB Community Health Care NHS Trust:
Minara Karim
Ethnic Services Co-ordinator
BHB Community Health Care NHS Trust
Suttons View
St George's Hospital
117 Suttons Lane
Hornchurch
Essex RM12 6RS
Telephone: 01708 465389

Broadmoor Hospital Authority:
Tony Lingiah
Professional Development Adviser
Broadmoor Hospital
Crowthorne
Berkshire RG45 7EG
Telephone: 01344 754408

Community Health Care Service North Derbyshire NHS Trust:
Sandra Mitchell
Confederation Director for Mental Health
Community Health Care Service North Derbyshire NHS Trust
Walton Hospital
Whitecotes Lane
Chesterfield
Derbyshire S40 3HN
Telephone: 01246 551785

Dudley Priority Health NHS Trust:
Miss Jane Bakewell
General Manager for Mental Health
Dudley Priority Health NHS Trust
Bushey Fields Hospital
Russells Hall
Dudley
West Midlands DY1 2LZ
Telephone: 01384 457373

Guild Community Healthcare NHS Trust:
Charles Flynn
Director of Clinical Services
Guild Community Healthcare Trust
Moor Park House
1 Moor Park Avenue
Preston PR1 6AS
Telephone: 01772 401010

Kneesworth House Psychiatric Hospital:

Frank Corr
Patient Services Director
Kneesworth House Psychiatric Hospital
Bassingbourn-cum-Kneesworth
Royston
Hertfordshire SG8 5JP
Telephone: 01763 255700

Northampton Community Healthcare NHS Trust:

Ms Sue Haynes, Patient Services Manager, Acute Inpatients
Telephone: 01604 752323

North Manchester Healthcare NHS Trust:

Mrs M Worsley
Divisional Director of Mental Health
North Manchester Healthcare NHS Trust
Delauneys Road
Crumpshall
Manchester M8 5RL
Telephone: 0161 720 2424

North Warwickshire NHS Trust:

Christine Trethowan
North Warwickshire NHS Trust
139 Earls Road
Nuneaton
Warwickshire CV11 5HP
Telephone: 01203 642200

Northwest Anglia Healthcare NHS Trust:

Stuart Hatton, Director of Mental Health and Learning Disability Services
Telephone: 01733 318110

Portsmouth Health Care NHS Trust:

Lesley Humphrey
Quality Manager
Portsmouth Health Care NHS Trust
St James' Hospital
Locksway Road
Portsmouth
Hants PO4 8LD
Tel. 01705 822444

Shap Working Party on World Religions in Education:
Mike Berry
Shap Co-ordinator
c/o The National Society's RE Centre
36 Causton Street
London SW1P 4AU
Tel. 020 7932 1194

St Andrew's Hospital:
Dr Marie Midgley
Quality Assurance Co-ordinator
St Andrew's Hospital
Billing Road
Northampton NN1 5DG
Telephone: 01604 629696

Wolverhampton Health Care NHS Trust:
as before

Provision and use of interpreters

Barnet Healthcare NHS Trust:
Raj Guzhadhur, Ethnic Monitoring Manager
Telephone: 020 8732 6454

Ealing, Hammersmith and Fulham NHS Trust:
as before

Lambeth, Southwark and Lewisham Health Authority Interpreting Service:
Satinder Alg
Interpreting Service Manager
Lambeth Southwark and Lewisham HA
1 Lower Marsh
London SE1 7NT
Telephone: 020 7716 7056

Language Indicator Prompt System (Lips):
Brian Payne
Commissioning Manager
London Borough of Haringey Social Services Department
40 Cumberland Road
Wood Green
London N22 4SG
Telephone: 020 8489 3914

Language Line:
Jon O'Keefe
Public Sector Sales Director
Language Line
Swallow House
11-21 Northdown Street
London N1 9BN
Tel. 020 7520 1430

Northampton Community Healthcare NHS Trust:
as before

North Warwickshire NHS Trust:
as before

North West Anglia Healthcare NHS Trust:
as before

Rampton Hospital Authority:
James Pam
Professional Head of Social Work Services
Rampton Hospital Authority
Retford
Notts DN22 0PD
Telephone: 01777 248321

South London and Maudsley NHS Trust:
Zoe Reed
Director of Organisational and Community Development
South London and Maudsley NHS Trust
Leegate House
Burnt Ash Road
Lee Green
London SE12 8RG
Telephone: 020 8297 0707

Thames Gateway NHS Trust:
as before

REFERENCES

[1] The Sainsbury Centre for Mental Health (1997) *The National Visit. A one-day Visit to 309 Acute Psychiatric Wards by the Mental Health Act Commission in collaboration with The Sainsbury Centre for Mental Health.*

[2] Department of Health (1994) *Collection of ethnic group data for admitted patients.* EL(94)77.

[3] Department of Health (1994) *Collecting ethnic group data for admitted patient care. Implementation guidance and training material.* NHS Executive.

[4] Davies S., Thornicroft G., Leese M., Higgingbotham A. & Phelan M. (1996) Ethnic differences in risk of compulsory psychiatric admission among representative cases of psychosis in London. *British Medical Journal* **312** (7030) 533-7.

[5] Littlewood R. & Lipsedge M. (1993, 2nd edition) *Aliens and Alienists.* London: Routledge.

[6] Department of Health (1999) *Tackling Racial Harassment in the NHS – A Plan for Action.* HSC 1999/060.

[7] Warner, L. and Ford, R. (1998) Conditions for women in inpatient psychiatric units: the Mental Health Act Commission 1996 National Visit. *Mental Health Care* **1** (7) 225-228.

[8] The Sainsbury Centre for Mental Health (1997) *Pulling Together: The future roles and training of mental health staff.*

[9] Department of Health (1999) *National Service Framework for Mental Health. Modern Standards and Service Models.* The Stationery Office.

[10] Mental Health Act Commission (1999) *Eighth Biennial Report 1997-1999.* The Stationery Office.

[11] Department of Health and Welsh Office (1999) *Mental Health Act 1983 Code of Practice.* The Stationery Office.

[12] Mental Health Act Commission (1985) *First Biennial Report 1983-1985.* HMSO.

NOTES